A "One Evening" Condensed Book

The HEALING of PERSONS

By Paul Tournier M.D.

Published by
GOOD NEWS PUBLISHERS
Westchester, Ill. 60153

Foreword

When Dr. Tournier told me how disturbed he had been, in the course of ten years' medical practice, by the insufficiency of classical and official medicine as regards certain chronic diseases, and how he had gradually become convinced that in many cases what mattered was the eradication of the psychological causes of the condition rather than the correction of its passing corporeal manifestations, I could not but encourage him wholeheartedly to devote himself to the task to which he felt called.

According to their attitude of mind or the advice of those around them, some patients turn to psychoanalysis or to Christian Science, which often brings them momentary relief, but which will not procure for them the definitive liberation that alone can lead to the individual and total solution of what Dr. Tournier rightly calls "personal problems," problems that are raised for all sincerely thinking persons among us. With fine courage and fervor, Dr. Tournier makes a frontal attack on these personal problems. His excellent book provides striking examples of this on every page. All who read this book, both doctors and patients, must congratulate the author for having put his encouraging experiences within the reach of everyone.

Georges Bickel
Professor in the Faculty of Medicine
Geneva, Switzerland

Preface

I recently treated a young woman who had undergone a very well-conducted course of psychoanalysis lasting a number of years.

She was a Christian, and had even been an active propagator of her faith. She suffered, however, from psychological difficulties, and she had at last been forced to recognize that she was using her faith to hide from herself the fact that she had a number of unsolved problems in her life and in her heart.

One day I saw that young woman come to me and ask me only to be the silent witness of her confession, the confession of a wrongdoing which, throughout the duration of the analysis, had weighted on her life without her being delivered from it. And I saw her rise, radiant.

I mention this case because it seems to me to illustrate the truth that men's problems are at one and the same time infinitely complex and exceedingly simple—complex from the technical point of view, and simple from the spiritual point of view; and also because I have heard, to my great surprise, that several readers of this book have thought it possible to conclude from it that I denied the complexity of men's physical and psychological problems. Nothing is further removed from my mind and my experience.

If my book encourages sick people to talk more confidently to their physician about the secret wounds festering in their hearts, they will find his help more effective. And their experiences will fill better than I could the gaps in its pages.

There is, however, one question which many readers have addressed to me and which I cannot omit to mention here: "Does it last? What has happened in the long run to the patients of whom you write?"

I can only say that the spiritual life is no different from everything else in this world: No step forward is maintained unless it is followed by further steps. He who does not go forward, goes back. Physical, psychical, and spiritual health is not a haven in which we can take refuge in a sort of final security, but a daily battle.

P. T.

Medicine and Life

"Man does not die," a doctor has remarked. "He kills himself."

God has a purpose for our life, as for the world. And if the world is sick today because it is disobeying God's laws, men too are sick because they do not live in accordance with God's purpose. So the highest role of the doctor is to help men to discern what is God's purpose for their lives and to conform therewith.

Every act of physical, psychological, or moral disobedience of God's purpose is an act of wrong living, and has its inevitable consequences. Moreover, it does not compromise only the health of the person who commits it, but also that of other persons, and that of his descendants.

"Treat the patient, not the disease." Such is the precept our masters teach us, and which we are reminded of every day by medical practice. Take two patients suffering from the same disease: One makes a rapid recovery, while the other is handicapped by some secret worry which has destroyed his will to live. But to treat the patient and not the disease means penetrating into these personal problems, which our patients often hide from us in order to keep them hidden from themselves.

I remember a young woman who was not one of my patients, but with whom both my wife and I had profound discussions on religious matters.

The child of divorced parents, beset by tremendous difficulties that stemmed from her mother's nervous state, imbued with a lively faith, but wild, independent, and critical, she too reacted by tensing herself against adversity. For many years she overworked, sleeping only a few hours every night, and cutting down on food in order to meet her financial burdens, in spite of the first signs of failure in her general condition.

And when the lung infection revealed itself, she accepted it with all her usual pluck, but without throttling her lively and independent spirit, and filled with pride when by some subterfuge she could disobey the doctor's orders.

As soon as she felt a little better she longed to return to an active and adventurous life, and accepted the demands of her treatment only in the hope of enjoying the compensations that such a future would afford.

I brought to this sick girl the Christian message of total acceptance of disease and abdication before God of all self-will.

Just as my wife and I were leaving her room she called us back to say, in a voice that was filled with emotion: "You are right, what I need is to abdicate more thoroughly. I knew God was asking me to take some fresh step, but I did not know what it was."

Some time afterward she wrote to us: "I have truly accepted my illness—its spiritual as well as its physical suffering. There is no rebellion left in me. God has given me such peace that people have been asking what is the cause of the change that has taken place, and that has given me an opportunity to witness to my faith...."

I do not need to dwell on the influence of personal problems on those who suffer from the arthritic group of diseases. In these patients a large number of factors are mixed up together. First, there are the hereditary factors—one might say that what may be called the "arthritic terrain" is traceable to wrong modes of life of previous generations; and second, personal factors, both physical and moral.

Among wrong physical modes of life, alongside overwork and lack of exercise, wrong eating plays an important part: diets that contain too much meat or too many sweet foods, or that are too acid; or overuse of alcohol—in short, diets governed by gluttony. In God's plan of creation there is a proper diet for man, and man cannot neglect it with impunity.

I know one such patient whose doctor, aware of the part played by the psyche in her liver troubles, had recommended that she seek relaxation. For relaxation she listened to the radio. Unfortunately the radio is not always soothing. And when this patient, who nursed in her heart a keen resentment against certain foreign statesmen, chanced to hear them making speeches on the radio, she was so upset by it that another attack of her liver complaint was the result. It is clear that the true solution would have been found not in "relaxation," but in being set free from all the resentment that was poisoning her mind.

Every doctor could give any number of examples of this kind from his own experience.

The same thing could be demonstrated in the case of phlebitis, which usually occurs in subjects who are physically and morally fatigued. I am thinking of a patient who was immobilized for several months by phlebitis. It was followed by pneumonia, a sure sign of the weakening of his powers of resistance. Nevertheless, the pneumonia healed rapidly, and the patient was convalesing very satisfactorily when the phlebitis recurred. This happened just when he was having a serious disagreement with his employer, who was thinking of dismissing him because of his long illness. Everyone knows the strain caused by situations such as this.

It would be very interesting to conduct systematic research into the moral problems of those who suffer from chronic skin diseases. The patient care of the doctor achieves some betterment, and then all at once, just when the victory seems to have been won, and without any obvious cause, there is a recurrence and within a few hours the skin erupts again. It is only rarely that the patient will reveal to the doctor what is happening in his inner life at such moments.

I am called to an old lady of eighty-six who has tachycardia, a state which cannot be classed as a cardiac neurosis. We shall call her Felicienne. On her table is a bottle of digitalis, prescribed some days before by a Poor Law doctor. She confesses that she has taken three times the amount of the prescribed dose, in the hope that it would work better! Thinking that she has had enough digitalis, I put her on quinidine and give instructions that all excitement must be rigorously avoided.

On my next visit I find her heartbeats quite regular, and put it down to the beneficial effects of the quinidine. But I have the curiosity to ask my little old lady, now that she is easier to talk to, if there is perhaps some moral factor behind her heart attack. She at once exclaims: "There is indeed! They killed my cat! And it was on that very day that my palpitations started!" She had taken good care not to mention the fact to the first doctor, who would perhaps have prescribed a modest sedative instead of digitalis.

I have wished simply by means of examples to show the importance of personal problems. If this is so great in the case of patients suffering from organic diseases, it is even greater in those afflicted by functional and psychical disturbances.

The terror of past centuries was the scourge of great epidemics such as cholera, plague, smallpox, and puerperal fever. In this field, the success of medicine is a veritable triumph. Unhappily, a new specter menaces humanity today—its nervous state. The number of minor psychopathic conditions, of functional disturbances, of neuroses and psychoses has increased catastrophically over the last hundred years. This increase, says Dr. Alexis Carrel, can be "more dangerous for civilization than infectious diseases." Again, he says that "mental diseases by themselves are more numerous than all the other diseases put together.

He senses that patients are not so much diseased as the victims of the physical and moral disorders of their own lives and those of the set in which they move. They have more need of advice than of remedies, but do not follow the advice he gives them. What they need is to find a spiritual axis for their lives rather than any sort of medical treatment.

He realizes that the increase in the number of nervous complaints is due to a general moral recession. This recession, in fact, with its consequences in family, professional, and social life, increases the number of problems that are due to marital, family, and social conflicts, to emotional shocks, to uncertainty and fear, to the falling off in honesty and trust, to worry and immorality.

Of these sufferers from nervous complaints, most are women, for it is the social and moral position of women that has undergone the most radical change during the last half-century. When, of old, a woman was married by her parents to a man whom she did not love; when she was the victim of the egotism and authoritarianism of a husband to whom she was a domestic servant, and who was unfaithful to her, she did indeed suffer, but she ac-

11

cepted her lot because the social conventions offered her no hope of escape. Nowadays she can contemplate divorce. And from the moment the idea occurs to her, her sufferings seem more unbearable, her conflicts with her husband become more serious, so that she finishes up suffering more acutely still. In a society governed by undisputed moral principles, life was relatively simple; their collapse increases the number of moral "problems" in face of which the individual is left bewildered and powerless.

I wish to be very careful to avoid all misunderstanding on this subject. We must not look for the restoration of social conventionalism which was often moral only on the surface. This formalism of principles, even when it appeared to accord with Christian teaching, was too much imbued with the spirit of the Pharisees, against which Christ inveighed with the utmost rigor.

But Formalism is not Christianity. One might even say that it is essentially the negation of it. It was what crucified Christ. So then, if in this book I state my conviction that what the world and medicine stand most in need of today is a moral and spiritual renewal, this does not mean that I am advocating a return to the formalism of the beginning of the century, but rather the building of a new civilization in which the spirit of Christ will be the inner source of personal, family, social, and individual conduct.

The reader may object, however, that everybody comes up against difficulties in life—disappointments, remorse, injustice, conflicts—but everybody does not fall ill. The truth is that we all experience functional disturbances in varying degrees of intensity and persistence. If we examine closely the psychological reactions which are interfering with the normality of behavior in a neurotic, we are compelled to recognize that they are not of a different kind from our own, but merely more intense: They are still fear, jealousy, susceptibility, anger, dissimulation, self-pity, sentimentality, erotic desire, and depression. What characterizes the neurotic is the fact that the very intensity of his reactions sets up a vicious circle from which he is unable to escape on his own. His fear, for example, destroys his self-confidence, and his lack of confidence feeds his fear. He is afraid of himself, afraid of being ill, and it is this fear which is making him ill. The psychoanalysts have demonstrated that all the unconscious reactions of neurotics may be observed in the daily life of healthy persons. I entirely share their views on the continuity between the normal and the pathological in the case of psychoneuroses. All the behavior traits of the neurotic may be seen in our own false reactions to the problems of our lives. One goes a considerable way toward helping these sufferers in showing them frankly that one has reactions similar to theirs, since this takes away from them their feeling of isolation in being different from other people.

As a result of an insult, an injustice, a disappointment, we suffer from insomnia, anxiety, palpitations, displacement of affect, or overcompensation. In any case, these motor responses constitute a sort of self-treatment, an emotional discharge. Everyone knows that weeping brings relief. By means of this motor response, and also through the effect of the passing of time and through the instinctive forces of life and balance "gaining the upper hand," the reaction is gradually diminished. This is what I shall call the "minor liquidation" of the shock received, for rather than really healing it, it covers over the wound, to which the subject becomes resigned.

It is in fact by means of this "minor liquidation" that we neutralize by far the greatest number of our emotional shocks. But there is another course, which

I shall call "major liquidation." It is the spiritual way. If we bring an insult or a disappointment to God, we can be delivered from it. What takes place then is a true liquidation, for then hate gives way to love, rebellion to acceptance.

If one looks closely into it, one realizes that there is no disease, however "physical," so to speak, which is not complicated with an element of neurosis. In her book *Servitude et grandeur de la maladie,* Mme. France Pastorelli makes a penetrating analysis of the psychological complexes which are inevitably set up between the patient and those around him—the family, the nurse, and the doctor—and which can be resolved only on the spiritual level. It is impossible completely to avoid all affectation when faced with a sick person, whether it be the harshness of incomprehension, sentimental commiseration, calculated optimism, worried pessimism, veiled irritation, or helplessness. And the trouble is that every failure to act naturally brings into being an element of neurosis, which in its turn compromises the treatment and inhibits spontaneity.

My own experience is that in following Christ one can learn to act naturally once more. He pointed this out himself when he said that in order to enter the kingdom of God one had to become like a child. It is characteristic of the child that he is natural. He can be natural even with people who are not acting naturally, and whom he thus helps to be natural again.

In communion with Christ the person suffering from nerves can rediscover the childlike mind, simple and uncomplicated; he can break the vicious circles of fear and rancor, and dare to show himself to others as he really is, without hiding his weaknesses.

In communion with Christ the doctor steps down from his scientist's pedestal, approaches his patient man to man, and is enabled to act naturally toward him.

14

The Knowledge of Man

The whole sense of this book is to show that a "medicine of the person" is made up of two methods. The scientific teaching of the medical faculty prepares the doctor well for the analytical study of the physicochemical, physiological, and psychological phenomena of man. There can be no question of doing without these techniques. I have often been consulted in recent years by students desirous of fitting themselves to practice a medicine of the person. I have always urged them to acquire during their years of medical training the most thorough scientific grounding the university can provide. But the doctor who wants really to understand men must add to this knowledge an experience of a spiritual nature. As Duhamel wrote, the doctor's art is essentially a "singular colloquy with the sick person," a confrontation of two men who can really understand each other on a spiritual level.

Man is not just a body and a mind. He is a spiritual being. It is impossible to know him if one disregards his deepest reality. This is indeed the daily experience of the doctor. No physiological or psychological analysis

15

is sufficient to unravel the infinitely complex skein of a human life. He sees how little his patients understand themselves, as long as they do not examine themselves before God; how apt they are to close their eyes to their own faults; how their good will is held back by circumstances, discouragement, and habit; how little effect his advice can have in reforming a person's life when the patient's mind is torn by an inner conflict.

When I decided to devote all my energies toward acquiring this deep knowledge of man, the first precondition seemed to me to be the necessity of giving more time to each of my patients, and in order to do so, to accept a smaller number. The way our profession has developed has had the effect of turning the modern doctor into a man in a hurry. Many of my colleagues suffer from the sort of life they have to lead, in which too many patients troop through their consulting rooms, generally without leaving the doctors time enough really to get to know them. The development of social welfare plans and the standardization of doctors' fees have largely contributed to this state of affairs, which is one that must be put right.

The result is that patients see their doctors very frequently—or even a large number of doctors—without ever having time to seek the hidden cause behind the ills they suffer from. The diagnosis is arrived at after a clinical or radiological exploration, or a laboratory investigation. The patients are given advice and medicines. They recover successively from a number of illnesses. But why their resistance is weakened, why they have so many diseases in succession, why they lack the strength to live as they ought to live in order to be in good health, they only rarely have time to go into with their doctors.

To understand a person's life, to help him to understand it himself, takes a long time.

A thing that had struck me in the Paris hospitals was the consummate art with which the Masters, the heirs of the best French clinical traditions, conducted the interrogations of their patients. These interrogations were long and profound, always throbbing with human interest, full of penetrating insights into the drama of human life. They knew how to "make the patient talk," or to cajole him into a feeling of confidence so that he would say what was on his mind, in his own often very expressive language. Such interrogations often sufficed to enable the doctor to make a firm diagnosis—and he never failed to underline this with a slightly disdainful remark to the effect that the "gentlemen in the laboratory" could not but confirm it.

But these interrogations often went beyond the diagnosis and gave the complete outline of a person's life, showing where things had gone wrong, throwing a searching light on the secret problems that had played a decisive part in the development of the disease.

There was the case of Ginette. I was called in for an ordinary condition, and observed a pronounced curvature of the spine which the school doctor had already noted, and for which he had sent her to an orthopedist who had had a leather corset made for her. Radiography showed that there was no lesion in the vertebral column. The doctor had said to her: "You hold yourself badly; you must straighten yourself up. You see, we are forced to fit an appliance on you so as to stop your lungs from being compressed all the time."

I had a talk with her mother, intrigued by the question as to why the child should stoop like that.

I learned that the parents got on together very badly. The father was in the habit of causing noisy scenes at home. Not content with taking it out on his wife, he bullied his children, and the little girl was terrified of him. She no longer dared to speak to him, and withdrew into a corner like a hunted beast.

I realized then that the physical attitude of the girl was but the reflection of her moral attitude of fear. Instead of developing happily as a child of her age should, holding her head high and breathing deeply, she shrank into a worried stoop. Look at people whom you know, and see how their attitude, their gait, and their way of standing and sitting reflect their state of mind.

All these false attitudes, these bodies which stoop because their minds are closed up, have more influence on health than we think, on the intensity of the respiratory process, on physical vitality and resistance to disease. They will not, however, be corrected merely by the use of leather corsets, exhortation, or even by physical exercises. They call for a doctor who, in addition, concerns himself with the solution of the personal problems of the patient's life.

The work of psychoanalysts has provided many other illustrations of this symbolization of the mind by the body. This is the "meaning" of the symptoms of neuroses. A hysterical paralysis is the materialization of a refusal to move forward in life.

In the same way body and mind are a symbol of the soul, of a man's attitude to God.

But while the study of the body and the mind is pursued along analytical, technical, and objective lines, that of the spiritual being eludes all extrinsic investigation. It is for this reason that it is the key to a synthesized knowledge of man.

God has a purpose for every man. To live in accordance with this purpose is man's normal life. To depart from it physically, morally, or spiritually is what I have called "wrong living," which has harmful repercussions on health. The task of the doctor, therefore, is to help men to see what is God's purpose for their lives, so that they may succeed in living the lives that are normal for them.

18

There is a mixture in a person's temperament of factors which come from God and factors which derive from wrong living. By means of prayer and meditation a man can distinguish what things in his temperament are God-given, and must be accepted, from what comes from wrong living and must be corrected.

The study of temperaments opens up interesting perspectives into what might be called the medicine of the healthy.

"Prevention is better than cure," people say. And yet doctors rarely see the healthy. Most people go to the doctor only when they are afraid: afraid of disease, of infirmity, or of death. I have had an increasing number of physically healthy people coming to see me over the last few years. Their motives in coming to consult me were quite different. For the love of God, out of a desire to obey him and to devote to his service the best of their health, strength, and talents, they were seeking to know themselves better, so as to organize their way of living, their food, and their rest in accordance with his will. It is a great joy to the doctor to be able to help a healthy person in this way to make himself even healthier, and to improve his usefulness to society. It is, in a way, to help him to build up positive health: not a health whose sole aim is to help him to avoid disease, but one that will help him to render better service. It is a great joy too for the doctor sometimes to meet a well-built man, full of possibilities. In our study and practice we hardly ever see a normal man.

The choleric—energetic and domineering, imagining little but achieving much, seeing things as black and white rather than in shades of gray, insensitive and hard-hearted, but leading a life of toil as severe on himself as on others, preferring quantity and speed to quality and depth—finds himself quite at home in this technological civilization. He occupies the positions of authority in political, economic, and even intellectual life, and imposes his faster temperamental rhythm on the social machine.

And so it is from among the sensitive, the artistic, the phlegmatic types that this society recruits its social misfits. The choleric sets the tone, and the conscientious but passive phlegmatic looks like a failure.

But in making men different, God meant every man to have his equal place in society, and the present crisis in our civilization demonstrates that this elevation of the man of action to the rank of social norm can lead only to an impasse. All our effort and activity, all our standardization and organization end in political, economic, and psychological crises without precedent.

Creative imagination, calm thought, artistic production, the gentle things of life, the things of the heart and the soul have been strangled in this race to achieve and produce more and more. And humanity has no idea what to do with all its material wealth and all the products of its activity. It suffers from sterility amidst its granaries. It has looked for profits and can no longer even sell. For in a civilization in which action and technical progress have become the norm, money is king, and material return the only criterion of value.

And our mental hospitals are filled with people whose natures are artistic, gentle, and intuitive, crushed by the struggle to live, incapable of keeping up with the speed of the men of action, incapable of earning their living, defeated by the wounds inflicted on their sensitivity, stultified by their feelings of inferiority and social uselessness, discouraged and lacking faith in themselves. For though the phlegmatic is passive he is by no means insensitive—quite the contrary.

So then, man's temperament is a factor which, like everything he possesses, is neither good nor bad in itself. Each temperament has its dangers: authoritarianism in the choleric, negativism or gluttony in the lymphatic, falsehood or day-dreaming in the sanguine, and egoism in the melancholic. Each temperament has also its treasures.

The reason for our study of temperaments is that we may learn better to know ourselves and what God wants of us. It is in order to submit and consecrate our temperament to God, for him to use in accordance with his purpose.

Look anywhere in the Gospel story and you will see that those whose lives were decisively transformed through their contact with Christ belonged to the most varied categories of temperament: the shy and the impulsive, the humble and the proud, the practical and the intellectual. Alongside them, people of all classes of temperament—and among them, be it noted, many theologians fond of religious arguments—were able to brush past Christ without having any religious experience at all. They saw and heard the same things, which got no further than the surface of their minds, and were never integrated into life. Therefore, though in this book I stress the medical importance of a true decision for Christ, I am careful not to confuse it with a sentimental inclination toward religion.

One might similarly think at first sight that confession would come more easily to an extrovert than to an introvert. The former, with his easy jovial manner, readily talks about himself. "The thing about me, " he says,"is that I hide nothing. If anything, I am too frank." But this is a more apparent than real self-revelation. It leads to no spiritual experience so long as it does not get beyond the flood of easy confidences to the thin trickle of real confessions. The problem of the human heart is the same for each of us, and is independent of character. The road to Christ is not easier for some than it is for others. It is difficult for all.

In the same way also optimism can be mistaken for faith. I am by nature optimistic, whereas my wife is pessimistic. I am confident, she is apprehensive. For a long time I reproached her for her pessimism as indicating lack of faith. For my own part I prided myself on my optimistic outlook as if it came from my faith and not from my inborn disposition. One day, when we both had a great act of faith to perform, I realized during my quiet time that I was being less than honest in confusing faith and optimism, to my own advantage. The truth was that real faith was as difficult for me as it was for my wife. And so I was much better able to help her to overcome by faith her natural pessimism than when I used to contrast it with my thoughtless optimism. It helped me also to see what it was that was making my Christian witness sterile as far as timid, skeptical, and pessimistic people were concerned. For as long as they felt that in what I said about faith there was more of natural optimism than of real faith, they tended to think that that was "all right for confident people," but that it was not for them.

The study of temperament ought to help us to live in accordance with our own true nature, to cultivate the talents which God has shared out to us, instead of comparing ourselves with other people, envying their gifts and being thrown into despair because we feel inferior to them. God loves each person equally and knows well that no one man is more valuable than another.

It is of course between husband and wife that this mutual comparison is most frequently made and is most dangerous. For it leads to a progressive accentuation of the dominances of each temperament, which may eventually lead to what it is fashionable to call "incompatibility of temperament." Perhaps I may be permitted once more to make myself clear by quoting my own experience, since this psychological phenomenon is not the monopoly of marriages that are "on the rocks"; it is found in the happiest families. The more apprehensive my wife became, the more I tried to counterbalance her fears by adopting an air of confidence, even overdoing it sometimes, in order to cover up my own fears, for fear of encouraging hers. But the more confident I showed myself, the more my wife expressed her fears, in order to save me from falling into culpable overconfidence. The more advice she gave to the children, the more silent I became. And the more silent I was, the more advice she gave. One day she complained to me about my silence, and in my quiet time I saw that my behavior, instead of being regulated by a desire to obey the will of God, was in fact controlled by my natural temperament and my wish to counterbalance that of my wife. There was nothing to stop this vicious circle from growing worse and worse, unless it was broken by a change of attitude. And I saw at once that if I were to take my own responsibility toward the children more seriously, my wife would be able to sit more lightly to hers. Medical experience has taught me that there is no home that escapes this law of conjugal counterbalance. It manifests itself in a thousand different ways—loquacity and silence, expansiveness and reticence, optimism and pessimism, intellectualism and materialism, vivacity and gentleness, a love of solitude and a liking for society, conventionality and fantasy. It lies at the root of countless personal problems, or at least exacerbates them; and it can lead to well-nigh insoluble marital conflicts.

Among all the personal problems to which I have made it my purpose to refer in this book, there is no doubt that there are none which have more importance for the physical and psychological health of mankind than marital conflicts.

The mystery of sex is generally the first thing to make a breach in the complete confidence existing between children and parents and to erect moral barriers between them. It is often because they have not found the solution of their own sex difficulties that parents are embarrassed on this subject in front of their children and incapable of giving them a good sex education. Sometimes their complete silence leaves the child a prey to unhealthy curiosity, and often to exhausting masturbation, followed by precocious sexual abuses. In this way young people, through having made a bad beginning in their sex life, spoil their happiness forever. Sometimes, on the other hand, parents approach the subject in a spirit of conventional moralism which presents the whole subject of sex as sinful, says nothing of its divine aspect, sets up countless stubborn complexes, and plunges the young into a sterile and obsessive struggle against impurity which is as exhausting as sexual abuse, and undermines their confidence in themsleves.

And then there are all those unmarried people who never succeed in developing their personalities to the full because they never manage to come to terms with celibacy, while others, whether married or not, ruin their health in sexual excess. And there is the lifelong wearing down of physical and moral resistance by unreal imaginations, unhealthy reading, sexual selfishness, and the double life led by so many married people whom their guilty secret prevents from discovering the tonic force of true sexual harmony. The experience of the doctor shows him how few men and women there are who enjoy the physical and psychical powers which full and proper sexual development can bring.

Marital conflicts are even more difficult when it is the woman who is the stronger of the two. I mean strong not only in character but also in virtue. Among the couples who have come to me over the last few years, I could point to a large number whose problems are basically similar in outline.

Strong wives are thus constantly called upon to try and cope with the difficulties brought about by their husbands' weakness, acting in their place, paying their debts, and taking complete control, so that their lives are a continual burden.

Saint Paul remarks on how difficult the strong find it to understand the weak.

A miracle from God is needed. I have seen it happen in a sufficiently large number of cases to be able to affirm here that God has a solution to all these conflicts. But I have known also of sufficient failures not to underestimate the difficulties, and to know that apart from a miracle from God there is no answer to these marital vicious circles.

It is only when a husband and wife pray together before God that they find the secret of true harmony, that the difference in their temperaments, their ideas, and their tastes enriches their home instead of endangering it. There will be no further question of one imposing his will on the other, or of the other giving in for the sake of peace. Instead, they will together seek God's will, which alone will ensure that each will be able fully to develop his personality.

In every argument between a husband and wife there are apparent causes: conflicting ideas, opinions, ideals, and tastes. But behind these apparent causes there are real ones: lack of love, touchiness, fear, jealousy, self-centeredness, impurity, and lack of sincerity. Indeed, one may say that there are no marital problems; there are only individual problems. When each of the marriage partners seeks quietly, before God, to see his own faults, recognizes his sin, and asks the forgiveness of the other, marital problems are no more.

Most of all, a couple rediscovers complete mutual confidence, because, in meditating in prayer together, they learn to become absolutely honest with each other.

Such honesty is very difficult to achieve. One always feels that if one makes a total confession, if one reveals all one's secret thoughts, one must lose the confidence of one's partner forever. The truth is quite the contrary. A union founded on complete mutual frankness is notably more solid than one which is thought to be safeguarded by prudent reservations. This is the price to be paid if a man and a woman are to cease living side by side like strangers, to come out of their spiritual solitude and create a climate of normal mental life.

This is the price to be paid if partners very different from each other are to combine their gifts instead of setting them against each other.

Christianity consists in forgiving, forgiving even those who do not come to us and eat humble pie; and that following in Christ's footsteps, far from abasing us, on the contrary ennobles us.

I have not mentioned conflict between a child and an unjust teacher. But then I could not possibly list all the conflicts which spoil men's lives. There are all those connected with work—not only between employers and employees, but more often still between foremen and workmen, between jealous workmen, between competing employers. And there are all the social, political, and international conflicts. I do not need nowadays to emphasize the consequences of these on the lives and health of countless men, women, and children.

There, as in the family, only a return to God can bring a true solution—reconciliation between employer and employee, between competitors, between political opponents, between nations, and between races. I should be overstepping the limits of my book if I were to cite examples of this that are known to me.

Flight

Personal problems are interconnected like the links in a chain, that a matrimonial conflict, for example, may bring in its train rebelliousness, laxity, alcoholism, and dishonesty. For when a man does not feel strong enough, when he despairs of solving some vital problem in his life, he tries instinctively to conceal his defeat by running away. And this flight creates a new problem which makes setting right his life more difficult still. Sometimes he is aware of this, but more often the flight is unconscious.

There is, first, flight into dreams. Real life is harsh. It is constantly injuring our sensibilities. The temptation to escape from it by flight is the stronger the more sensitive we are: We run away in order to protect our sensitivity, to escape the conflict which wounds it. The land of dreams is close at hand, so that one can escape into it at any moment, far from these painful realities. The escape often takes the form of a continuous story, a novel in many episodes which a person tells himself, going over the episodes again and again, and which absorbs his mental energy. It is a secret treasure into which he pours the best of himself. It is his way of turning the tables on harsh reality. He composes for himself a life in which he is always winning victories, and this compensates for the defeats he sustains in real life. In his fantasy he always plays the star part, he is always loved, esteemed, understood; he is always in command, he is free to sacrifice himself nobly.

The sort of dream of which I am speaking here is sterile and ineffective. It is fatiguing rather than restful. Above all, it aggravates the divorce between the ideal and the real. We are the more ready to take flight on the wings of dreams the more mediocre reality is, and reality seems the more mediocre the more we compare it with some idealistic dream.

There is also flight into the past. Many people have their eyes turned constantly backward. They relive their Golden Age, a distant era in which they were happier, amid successes and joys. In this way they escape from the problems of the present, which they no longer try to solve, and savor the joys of the past.

Moreover, it is not only joys that are involved. Regret and remorse can act equally dangerously as a flight into the past. The scrupulous mind which is constantly going over the past, taking a somber pleasure in analyzing it, is escaping into unreality quite as surely as the one which goes back to its brighter pages. For the center of gravity of a person's life to be behind him is the opposite of true living, which is a march forward. Thus a person's existence becomes sterile and incapable of providing solutions for his problems.

And then there is flight into the future. Escaping into the future, constantly making plans, is another form of flight into dreams, another way of escaping from the imperfections of the present. In its extreme form it becomes what is called the flight of ideas. Thought follows thought in such rapid succession, jumping continually ahead, that they become ineffective, leading to no sustained action.

I used to have a tendency toward living in the future. I was always forming fresh projects which seemed to me to be finer than what I was engaged upon at the time. My wife, on the other hand, lived in the past. She only really enjoyed a journey after it was over, when she could be certain that no unforseen event would spoil it. Happily, we have met together in the present, to live truly together.

Living with God means living the present hour which he gives us, putting our whole heart into what he expects of us in that hour, and leaving the past and the future to him, to whom they belong.

The reader will have some idea of how much might be said about flight into disease. The fact is too common and well-known for me to need to dwell on it. No one escapes it. Time and time again in my own case self-examination has shown that a sudden feeling of fatigue, a headache, or an attack of indigestion is really a trick played on me by my own unconscious. A difficulty or a disappointment had interrupted the smooth flow of my work; a difficult letter to write, a puzzling case to sort out, or a disagreeable task to be undertaken had held me up, and so my unconscious was furnishing me with a good excuse for postponing it. All functional disturbances and, *a fortiori,* all neuroses, may be seen to involve thus a secret flight into disease. This, of course, is not to say that the disease is therefore "imaginary." A serious injustice is done to people suffering from such disturbances if they are accused of inventing their troubles as an easy means of escape. The feeling of not being understood, of not having their troubles taken seriously, from which they so frequently suffer, prevents these people from coming out of their unconscious refuge. In order to be able to come out of the tiny shelter that they have built against the storms of life, they need to feel that they are understood, loved, and supported.

Mention must be made n o w of what may be called "noble flights." Addictions are not the only form of flight. Often some of the best things we do in this world are an escape.

I am thinking of art and of science. I know some scientists whose devotion to their work is wonderfully conscientious and fruitful. Nevertheless their work is a form of escape, compensation for a family life which is not a success. I am reminded of a man who told me that his life began when he went from his house to his artist's studio, and that it stopped again, in a sort of parenthesis, whenever he locked up his studio. How many studios a n d laboratories a c t in this way as an escape-world where we try to forget the reality outside which we do not know how to cope with?

I cannot close the list without referring to the most troublesome flight of all—flight into religion. The religious life itself can be an escape; an escape into a little mystic chapel which is like an island cut off from the world, where one can hide in order to escape the world and its wounds, to wallow in a passive enjoyment that is pointless and out of contact with reality. It is possible also to use the active and intellectual side of religion as an escape. I know myself how I have taken pleasure in theological arguments at which my mind was more flatteringly successful than it was in tackling the practical, concrete problems of my life.

Modern Western society is dominated and governed by noise, newspapers, radio, and speed, so that men have lost the sense of inner meditation, of mature reflection, and thoughtful action. But all this feverish activity is also a form of flight, by means of which men are trying to cover up the unease in their hearts, their spiritual emptiness, their defeats, and their rebellion.

A disciplined life in all spheres is one of the important conditions of physical and psychic health. Every day doctors have to deal with people who are worn out and unable to stand up to the life they lead. They generally assert that it is impossible to alter the way they live, and sincerely believe that their overwork is the product of circumstances, whereas it is bound up with their own intimate problems.

There seems to be a law of inertia in the psychological and physiological sphere, as there is in the realm of matter. On the one hand, a person who is run down may retain for a long time the appearance of health, while the balance of his strength is definitely in deficit. And on the other hand, when improvement in his condition begins he does not at first feel any amelioration. He retains a deceptive look of exhaustion which has to do largely with the destruction of his self-confidence. There is a sort of deferment of effect in both directions. It is as difficult to make a person who is overtaxing himself understand that the strength he thinks he has at his disposal is no longer anything but a facade as it is to make him realize, when he has cracked under the strain, that he could now take up some form of activity again, although he feels himself to be still in a state of exhaustion.

There are more intellectual and spiritual gluttons than one might think—that is to say, people who make excessive and undisciplined use even of the best things. I am thinking at the moment of a friend with whom I had conversations over a period of several months. He was a Jew. He was seeking Christ. But our long discussions were getting us nowhere. One day he came back to see me and told me he had found Christ. He had met a Christian who had simply told him that he was an intellectual glutton. Examining his conscience, he had suddenly seen that his inexhaustible religious discussions, how-

31

ever interesting they might be, were nothing but a kind of intemperance, and that they were blocking the road to his conversion.

Speaking of God's purpose for the normal life of man, Carton formulates what he calls "the law of the three rests." First there is the annual rest, the example of which is given us by Nature, which rests during winter. It is possible that winter holidays are more beneficial than those taken in summer. At the time when insolation is such that we are deprived of part of the sun's energy, a few weeks in the mountains—in the snow with its strong ultra-violet irradiations—would without doubt be the best kind of holiday, and perhaps the day will come when the educational authorities will realize this. As early as the fifth century B.C. Hippocrates was recommending the reduction of activity and of food during the winter—he even prescribed only one meal a day!—in order to conform with the law of nature.

Next is the weekly rest, laid down in the Bible. Here again it is scarcely necessary to point out the constant misuse of Sunday, a day on which many people fatigue themselves even more than on weekdays.

Lastly there is the nocturnal rest, the importance of which was understood by Christ himself, and which our civilization has so drastically reduced with the perfecting of artificial lighting.

I need not stress the part played by worry, interior and exterior conflicts, temptations to impurity, fear, and ambition in this question of sleep.

I can remember my astonishment and even my indignation as a doctor, on hearing a lady remark, a few years ago, that insomnia was a symptom of sin. My experience of these last few years has led me to realize how much truth there is in this assertion. Doubtless there are exceptions, nor is the relation always direct; and it would be wrong to suggest that a person who sleeps well is less sinful than one who suffers from insomnia. But I cannot keep count of the number of patients I have seen rediscover the habit of sleep as a result of the transformation of their lives brought about by submission to Jesus Christ.

It is the quality of sleep which is changed as much as anything. Here is what one patient writes: "Sleeping less, I rest more, because my nights are absolutely calm now that my life belongs entirely to God. I sleep for about seven hours. Often less. I have learned to sleep in the afternoon when I have a moment's opportunity. My conviction is that God gives us complete directions for our physical life if we put ourselves entirely in his hands."

The opposite of flight into overwork is flight into passivity, withdrawal, negativism, and idleness.

Laziness has considerable importance in medicine. Many people, even apparently very active people, are lazy in that they exert themselves only as much as they find agreeable. Thus, for example, while engaging in intense intellectual activity they neglect, from laziness, all forms of physical exercise.

It is laziness which prevents so many people from rising early so as to have enough time for prayer before the day's work and entering upon it zealously and joyfully. It is laziness which ties up so many people in unsociable, narrow, distant lives, deprived of the continual social exchange which is the law of human life.

Lack of exercise is one of the commonest physical shortcomings. Its consequences on the health of the body are well known: obesity and plethora of the sedentary.

Order can of course be a personal problem, when it is so rigid and fussy that it is thought of as the most important thing in life. But disorder is also a problem, and one that is particularly harmful to the atmosphere of a person's life. I know something about this myself. I have a lot to do in this respect because I am untidy by nature. One day I saw that I had no right to suggest to others that they should put their lives in order when I myself had so many cupboards in disorder, letters unanswered, and unread medical journals piling up. When I said something of this to my son, he told me that he would pray that God would give me the strength and perseverance necessary for this great work. But on the following day he came back to talk to me about it. He had thought that he would help me even more by tidying up his own room to encourage me. Over a period of several months I gave up a number of other activities in order to get myself up to date, and it was a great liberation.

I want to say a word or two on silence. The effect on the nerves of modern man of immoderate use of the radio, of pneumatic drills, and of the noise of our big cities is well known. But modern man is afraid of silence, simply because of all the personal problems in his life which worry him and which he would like to forget. I know a theologian who had a serious secret problem and who always had his radio switched on when he was in his study, in order to avoid the silence in which the drama going on inside him became too acute.

Indiscipline is closely related to laziness and disorder. Charles was a man whom I got to know while he was unemployed. He had lost his job as a result of illness, and his heart was full of bitter resentment against social injustice. We had quite a lively discussion.

But three months later Charles, still unemployed, was in my consulting room again. He told me what had happened to him. During a walk in the mountains he had suddenly thought himself lost. At that moment the memory of the evening spent with me, and especially the memory of the serene joy of another unemployed man, had come to him. He had started to pray. His adventure ended without mishap, but as he came back down the mountain he had thought seriously over his own life. He was dissatisfied with himself and wanted to live the clear, confident life of which we had spoken. But he did not know how to go about it.

I told him what my own experience had been. Then he started to tell me of all the moral indiscipline to which the distress of unemployment had opened the door. I had a new man in front of me: no longer the victim blaming society, but the sinner acknowledging his own guilt. While he laid his faults before me one by one, I considered how great a moral danger the idleness of unemployment is for those who are lacking in culture and in depth of spiritual life. His wife, a militant Communist, had a job. And he, in his long empty day, could no longer even summon up enough energy to light the fire for dinner. His wife was threatening him with divorce, and their home was nothing but an arena for violent quarrels.

When he left me he said that he intended to get up early, begin his day with a period of meditation, and then take some exercise and do the housework.

His wife was astonished when, the next day at noon, she found the flat tidied up and the lunch ready.

He came back to see me and a friendship was formed between us. A few weeks later he was a quite different man, tidily dressed, disciplined, cheerful, and friendly. His home was happy and he soon found work.

At Christmastime I made the acquaintance of his wife. It was the first Christian festival she had taken part in since her childhood. She burst into tears when she heard her husband saying what God had done in his life and in his home. She made friends with my wife, and in her turn she unburdened herself to her.

One day two years later Charles came to me, very upset. He told me at once that he had been backsliding: that for some time he had given up meditation and prayer. And then temptations had come, and he had spent money which had been entrusted to him, and which he had now to pay back. He needed some money in order to get himself out of trouble. It was obvious what he had come for.

But I know that what he really needed was a fresh experience of God's grace, rather than to get off lightly. I told him calmly: "You are going to see your employer, Charles, and to tell him what you have done."

"But that means prison!" he exclaimed.

I chanced to meet him in the street next day. He was beaming. He came toward me eagerly. He had spent a terrible night, but he had finally been able to pray. His employer had received him quite differently from what he expected, and had proposed that he should pay the money back in monthly installments. Now he really was determined to be disciplined.

Suffering and Accepting Life

I propose to show now that the spiritual message of the Holy Scriptures is the only true answer to the problems of men's lives.

The Bible records the life and death of Jesus Christ, the God-man, who knew all our physical, psychic, and spiritual difficulties, and who alone, through his perfect obedience, resolved them all. He is the true Revelation; living in personal fellowship with him we see what our personal problems are, and above all we find the supernatural strength we need to supplement our own poor efforts to resolve them. Finally, through his sacrifice on the Cross, he brings us supreme deliverance, taking upon himself all the wrongs that our efforts have failed to put right, and granting us God's forgiveness.

The Bible alone gives a true answer to the incomprehensible mystery of suffering. To fight against suffering is to be on God's side. On the other hand suffering is often bound up with our disobedience and our wrong modes of life, so that in order to strive effectively against suffering we must bring souls to Christ, who delivers them from their faults, who in order to heal the paralytic said to him: "Your sins are forgiven" (Matt. 9:2).

Despite the most telling spiritual experiences, there subsist in every man's life sufferings which God does not relieve. So to St. Paul, who thrice asked God to remove his "thorn in the flesh," God answered: "My grace is sufficient for you" (II Cor. 12:9).

So the Christian answer to suffering is acceptance. Through acceptance, suffering bears spiritual fruit—and even psychic and physical fruit as well.

Resignation is passive. Acceptance is active. Resignation abandons the struggle against suffering. Acceptance strives without backsliding, but also without rebellion.

In a lecture delivered to the German Philosophical Society, the surgeon Sauerbruch declared: "Faith deeprooted in the soul has more efficacy than all philosophical knowledge. Pain and suffering find their liberating meaning only in the Christian faith. Christians see suffering as a means used by God to lead man along the holy road of affliction. An instrument for the purification and edifying of the Christian character."

A psychiatrist told me that he had once been summoned by an old friend whom he had not seen for a number of years, and who also had Parkinson's disease. The sick man had added to the message he sent: "Only come if you have some new remedy to bring. I've had enough of doctors who say they cannot cure me."

As he went into the bedroom the psychiatrist said to his friend: "I've brought you a new remedy—Jesus Christ."

His remark was not at all well received: The patient bitterly reproached his friend for mocking him. But when the psychiatrist had talked of the change brought about in his own life since he had encountered Jesus Christ, the tone of the conversation altered, and the patient opened his heart as well. This was the first of many conversations. The spiritual life of this patient was nonexistent. Up to then there had been no room in his mind for anything but rebellion against his illness. His friends, wearied by his complaining, came less and less often to see him. But now a real transformation was taking place. In spite of the drawn look which disease imparts to a face, his expression brightened and he looked years younger. Soon he found such peace that people came to him to share the mysterious strength they found in him.

Accepting suffering, bereavement, and disease does not mean taking pleasure in them, steeling oneself against them, or hoping that distractions or the passage of time will make us forget them. It means offering them to God so that he can make them bring forth fruit. One does not arrive at this through reasoning, nor is it to be understood through logic; it is the experience of the grace of God.

I had an old and dear friend, one of the men I have esteemed most highly. For some weeks his health had been deteriorating. It was on Christmas Day that the doctor who tended him asked me to go with him on what must be his last visit.

The patient could speak only with difficulty. Medicine could afford little relief; we concentrated on surrounding the sick man with our affection. I was left alone with him for a moment. He spoke painfully to me: "There's something I don't understand . . ." He did not succeed in saying what it was he did not understand. This struck me particularly in a man who all his life had been devoted to intellectual clarity. Faith had always had the last word with him, but it was allied to a most lively intelligence. One felt that he was still troubled by whatever it was he did not understand. But he was too weak now to put his problem into words. And I realized that it would have been useless to ask him any questions, or to start a discussion.

After a moment's silence, I bent over him and said quietly: "You know that the most important thing in this world is not to understand, but to accept." With a happy smile he stammered: "Yes . . . it's true . . . I do accept . . . everything." It was almost the last thing he said. After my visit he fell asleep. During the night he suddenly awoke, sat up, and said aloud: "I am going to heaven," and died.

The Christian message of acceptance is not an answer only to exceptional suffering. It applies to hundreds of different aspects of daily life. Acceptance of living is one of the most important factors in healing.

Lastly, acceptance of growing old means living in the present, at any age, even if the past has been rich in beautiful experiences. During a visit to one of my patients I admired the flowers on her balcony. But there were some faded flowers among them, and I said to her: "You must cut off the faded flowers so that the plant will grow new ones." I realized at once that this was a parable of life. The flowers were beautiful once, but time passes; and if we try to preserve the flowers of the past we have only faded flowers on our plant, and prevent it from producing new ones.

Parents, too, must accept their children. There are many parents who are disappointed in their children because the children do not fit into the fine pattern they had dreamed of. There are many children who feel vaguely oppressed by this undefined parental disapproval. Accepting one's children means accepting their temperaments, their failings, their character, and sex.

We cannot help others to find the strength to accept their lives if we have not found it ourselves. Only God gives it. Accepting one's life means accepting all that one considers to be unfair victimization, the injustices of fate as well as those of men. We sometimes say that we would be willing to accept the injustices provided that at least we were asked to forgive them. But the Christian is required to forgive even those who do not ask for forgiveness.

Accepting one's life means also accepting the sin of others which causes us suffering, accepting their nerves, their reactions, their enthusiasms, and even the talents and qualities by means of which they outshine us. It means accepting our families, our clients, our fellow workers, our place in society, our country.

Unless one has accepted one's work, one does it half-heartedly, and remains dissatisfied with the result. It is also much more tiring. I am reminded of a young woman who lost weight while at work, and put it on again during holidays, with astonishing rapidity. When we looked more closely into the situation we realized that what was damaging her health was not so much the work itself as the wearing effect of a constant revolt against that particular work.

Many people will not accept their own bodies. No one knows the secret torment, often childish, but capable of turning into a regular obsession, that can be caused by a nose that is too long, legs that are too thick, by being too tall or too short, by a tendency to plumpness, or an unharmonious voice—in short, by revolt against not being as handsome or as beautiful as one would like. What fixes these preoccupations, and makes them worse, is the very fact that they are secret; for very often if such worries were openly voiced, reassurance would be forthcoming from the person's friends, and he might be quite astonished to learn that his little physical defects are hardly noticed, and that his friends know how to appreciate his other and more important qualities.

Accepting one's physical make-up means that one will stop comparing oneself with others. My wife is delicate, while I am a man of action. One day during her meditation she came to see that God's purpose for her was different from his purpose for me. What he required from her was an account of her own talent, and not of mine. That was the beginning of a great development in her as a person.

Happiness, inner harmony, acceptance of our lives, the solving of conflicts with others, satisfaction in work, victory over sin, over idleness, and over selfishness have doubtless more influence on our vitality than all the other physical factors of diet, heredity, constitution, or rest. They constitute a sort of coefficient which multiplies the basic figure of physical vitality.

Acceptance of one's marriage partner brings us to the subject of sex. Acceptance of one's wife, as she is. Acceptance of one's husband, as he is.

Further, accepting one's marriage partner involves real acceptance of marriage itself. There are more married people than one would think who are not totally married, without any mental or emotional reservation, who do not accept the restrictions which marriage imposes on their liberty, their independence, their wish to go their own way and enjoy their own amusements and pleasures, and to spend their money as they like.

The first prerequisite of Christian marriage is that the man and the woman should have been brought together by God. I know a man who during his quiet time was guided to marry a girl who at the time meant nothing to him. His first reaction was negative. The idea seemed absurd: He did not even know what language she spoke. But about the same time the girl had a similar call, although she did not know that the man had had a similar experience. Their lives were soon united in love.

Next in importance is that the engagement should be in conformity with God's purpose. The happiness of many a marriage is spoiled by unchastity and selfishness during the period of the engagement.

Lastly, it is vital that the union should be submitted to the authority of God. Both partners must seek to establish spiritual communion. The dictates of the Scriptures should govern their attitude to each other, every difficulty being resolved through prayer. The home must find its meaning in service together of God.

There is nothing wrong with the sex instinct: What is sinful is its use outside what God meant it to be.

Without God, the regulation of the sex life in marriage is either a compromise in which each partner hides his real thoughts from the other, or else tyranny by one over the other, or it may be an artificial and rigid edifice of formal principles. No moral or psychological system can regulate by principles a domain which belongs to daily obedience to God, to the free submission to him of the conscience enlightened by the Scriptures and the teaching of the church. When God directs the sex life of a married couple, they can practice it divinely, if I may use the word—in a full mutual communion that is carnal, moral, and spiritual all at once. It is the crowning symbol of their total giving of themselves to each other.

Many parents and educators who generally have not themselves succeeded in resolving their own sex problems think they are helping young people by parading before them the specter of the supposedly terrible results of masturbation. These young people then get bogged down in a negative and obsessive struggle. They come to isolate this problem from all their other personal problems, such as that of having a frank and loving relationship with their parents. The reader must understand that I am not advocating here anything but a high ideal of purity in young people. But what I maintain is that the struggle for this ideal is effective only when it takes its place in the framework of a total consecration of one's life to Jesus Christ, and when obedience to him in all other respects concerns the young person quite as much as his sexual continence.

A positive struggle counts on the supernatural strength which Christ gives to those who dedicate the whole of their lives to him. I know a young man who when he was tempted, instead of bracing himself stiffly in a negative effort, used to get down on his knees and thank God for having placed in him such a life-force, and ask him how he ought to be using it.

The biblical message of acceptance is the only possible answer to the great problem of suffering.

From the miracles that are wrought through acceptance, it can be seen that spiritual strength is the greatest strength in the world. It can transform both peoples and individuals. It alone can ensure victory over the negative forces of selfishness, hate, fear, and disorder, which destroy peoples and undermine the health of individuals. It alone gives them the joy, energy, and zeal needed in the daily battle for life and for the defense of health.

Health is not the mere absence of disease. It is a quality of life, a physical, psychical, and spiritual unfolding, an exaltation of personal dynamism.

My aim in this book is not to write a treatise on psychology, nosology, philosophy, or theology, but to help us discover a new physical, psychical, and spiritual health, through submitting afresh to the sovereignty of God.

Inspiration and Confession

I have shown that the Bible is the surest source of information about God's plan for the lives of men. But it would be a serious misunderstanding of the wonderful message of Jesus Christ to see the Bible as no more than a collection of divine laws to which men ought to try to conform. This would be to fall into the error of legalism, formalism or moralism. Moral effort of this kind has nothing whatever to do with the miraculous transformation brought about by Christ in the person who opens his heart to him. The gospel is not a call to effort, but to faith.

Psychologists have clearly shown the futility of the idea that one can get rid of an obsession, regain confidence, or recall a forgotten name simply by trying harder. The fact that one can go to bed with a problem and "sleep on it," and wake up in the morning with the solution, is evidence of the beneficial effect of a relaxation of tension on the mental processes.

The person who makes tremendous efforts to become better is like a man pushing on a door marked PULL. He must relax his efforts before the door will open.

The Christian experience is the irruption of Jesus Christ into a person's life, bringing relaxation of tension, confidence, and a quite new liberating force, and abruptly changing the course of its development. Legalism, on the other hand, means slavery to "principles," and continual efforts to satisfy the imperious demands of a moral code.

True liberation through Jesus Christ, however, is a very rare thing. It is in order to hide from himself his lack of real experience that the religious person so often pretends to be freed from sins and passions from which he has not in fact been delivered. This lack of sincerity with himself sets up a conflict in him. The doctor sees plenty of these religious people, ravaged by inextricable inner conflicts. The man in the street does not need to be a psychologist to sense this fact, and he simply says that he has no desire to be like them.

Nothing is further from the spirit of Christ than exhorting a person sick in mind to make the effort of will of which he is incapable. On the other hand, to lead him into personal contact with Jesus Christ will be to help him to find the supernatural strength which will bring him victories his own efforts could never have won for him.

It is no light matter to struggle against sin! It is not sufficient to urge people to mend their ways, to point out the price that has to be paid for men's faults, to denounce the modern decline in moral standards, or to write impressive articles on the thirst for personal gain which has overtaken so many of our doctors. We underestimate the power of sin if we imagine that a few pointed books will provide a solution. There is no power that will stem the power of sin, apart from that of Jesus Christ himself. This is why leading a person to a personal encounter with Jesus, in prayer and meditation, is the only certain road toward a real transformation of his life.

Lives are not to be transformed by means of regulations and advice only; this merely tends to turn the regulations into a new tyranny laid on the backs of those who try to keep them. It is, above all, a misunderstanding of the nature of the tragedy in the heart of man: his powerlessness to conform to his own principles. "Incapable ourselves of doing any good thing," as Calvin said. If we are to become obedient to the will of God for us, we need something other than laws and exhortations. We must go through a real inner transformation. The source of all reformation of life is in personal fellowship with Jesus Christ.

This is why I feel that the deepest meaning of medicine is still not in "counseling lives," but in leading the sick to this personal encounter with Jesus Christ, so that accepting it they may discover a new quality of life, discern God's will for them, and receive the supernatural strength they need in order to obey it.

Advice acts from without. The spiritual revolution takes place within. When a man encounters Jesus Christ, he feels all at once that he has been freed from some passion or some habit to which he has been enslaved, from some fear or rancor against which he has deployed his stoutest efforts in vain.

Our modern world longs to rediscover the deep springs of life. It will succeed in finding them only by traveling along the road of the inner life which leads to the presence of God, the Creator of life.

In prayer and meditation we see quite simple things in our lives which our intelligence has failed to perceive. We are also inspired to act; for true life is made up of an alternation between meditation and action. They are complementary: meditation leads to action, and action is matured in meditation. This is the universal rhythm of withdrawal and advance, the inner life and the outward. Action prepared in meditation is quite different in quality from the hectic, breathless activity which characterizes our age, filling it with noise, agitation, and frenzy, and which is one of the chief causes of the catastrophic increase in the incidence of nervous diseases. We blame the railways, the automobile, the telephone, the radio, and the economic complexities of modern life. This is fair enough, but it is man who is really to blame.

For a long time I myself indulged in a restless kind of life, always racing the clock, always in a hurry, incapable of finding the time I needed for my spiritual life. Since I began devoting to it an average of an hour a day, and often longer, I have had to give up activities which I used to think essential. But I have found more happiness in my work, and have been able to put more into it.

One can spend one's whole life trying to obey God, conscientiously applying oneself, regularly and methodically, to the task; one can live a life of austerity and scrupulous uprightness, without ever knowing this explosion of joy, this quite new strength that bursts forth when one is face to face with God and says, Yes! to him with all one's heart.

The effect on one's health is considerable—directly, through the joy and the release of vitality which always accompany this decisive experience; and indirectly, through the solving of one's personal problems which it makes possible, and the harmonization of the whole personality.

There are certain functions in man's organism—the vegetative functions—which are not subject to his will. They are automatically subject, one might say, to the will of God. If, therefore, we disobey his will in the functions over which we have been given free control, discord results. It is as if in a beehive one section of the bees followed the divine purpose dictated to them by their instincts, while others departed from it. One might indeed describe such a hive as diseased.

This is why to seek in prayer the purpose of God for our lives, and to enjoy personal fellowship with Jesus Christ who delivers us from the things that stand in the way of that purpose, leads to that harmony of the whole person which is one of the prerequisites of health.

Christ himself compared this spiritual experience with the germinating seed. The seed contains potentially all the power which will develop as it grows, but the tree which will come from it is not yet manifested.

"I was nervous and high-strung," a young woman writes, "going rapidly from a period of enthusiasm to one of depression, always having ups and downs—tiring both to myself and to those I was with, and finding lack of sleep very hard to bear. My digestion was bad; I used to eat too quickly and was easily and often sick. I suffered from skin eruptions. I was a terrible glutton, and though I fought against it, it was without much success. I had very little self-control, and used to give way to all my feelings—anger, enthusiasm, or despair—not without a certain violence, in a way which was painful to the people about me. I began to pray, to obey; and my life began to be centered on Jesus Christ. . . .

"There came a day when I realized that a new balance had been established in my body—an evenness of temper. I hardly know now what it is to feel despairing and depressed. I feel tremendously joyful sometimes, but it is a deeper, calmer sort of joy. . . . I used to be ashamed of my sexual desires, which I restrained or not, as I could, and that was terribly painful to me and helped to give me a feeling of unbalance. . . . I can rest better now, too. The skin eruption has almost completely disappeared. My digestion is improved, and the vomiting hardly ever happens now. As for my gluttony, it has disappeared without trace, and without any effort on my part. I appreciate good food even more than before, without being tempted to eat too much of it. My sex life has become more balanced and mature. I used to hold myself badly before, too, and used to get backaches. I realized one day that I ought to do exercises every morning, and I was given the perseverance to keep it up; it has been a great help. My health is a personal testimony. But it has happened all by itself, I might even say without my knowing it. This new state of mine depends on my regular quiet times and my surrender to God. It isn't something acquired once and for all, but it remains and lasts in the measure to which I obey God, confess to him, and am freed from my sins. The health of my body depends upon the health of my soul."

What I have tried to emphasize in this chapter is that it is not the application of the laws of life that leads to Christ, but the personal encounter with Christ which transforms men's lives and helps them to return to the laws of life. It does not always require religious discourses to bring souls to this personal encounter. I may say that I only rarely take the initiative in starting conversations on spiritual matters. It is almost always my patients who broach the subject with me, because it is the point to which the exploration of personal problems always leads.

A friend of mine who was in great torment of mind went to see a certain young man. They spent almost the whole of the night talking together. My friend said: "I have so many problems to solve," and the young man answered: "There are no problems. There are only sins."

If I look honestly into my own heart, and into the tragic situation of humanity, which my vocation as a doctor allows me to do day after day, I see that behind all "personal problems" there lies, quite simply, sin.

It is in order to hide his own sin from himself that man has been so ready to welcome that positivist scientific outlook which denies sin. People no longer want to know about good and evil. . . . In place of strict principles, we have psychological explanations. Sin is rejected as one of those outworn ideas which in a century of intelligence ought to be dead and buried.

Christ's attitude to the problem of the connection between sin and disease is quite clear. First of all, he affirms that there is a connection when he says to the paralytic before healing him: "Your sins are forgiven" (Matt. 9:2). He indicates that his power to forgive sins and that of healing the sick are two different aspects of a single ministry. This unity between his spiritual action and his medical action strikes one all through the Gospel.

But on the other hand, when his disciples ask him about the man born blind (John 9:3) or the victims on whom the tower of Siloam fell (Luke 13:4), in an attempt to get him to formulate theologically, so to speak, this link between sin and the suffering of mankind, he categorically refuses to do so. Very clearly he wants to avoid the connection between sin and disease (which the whole of his ministry affirms) being used hypocritically to condemn the sick as specially sinful.

But he at once adds: "Unless you repent you will all likewise perish." In this way he brings them back to the consideration of their own sin. Christ calls men to recognize more clearly their own sin when they see the evils from which mankind suffers, and not to use these ills as the occasion for passing judgment on other people.

The fact is that in denying the reality of sin, by giving people to understand that a fault of character is due to the malfunctioning of an endocrine gland, or by calling some impure temptation a "psychological complex," science destroys man's sense of moral responsibility. The present state of the world shows where that leads.

Christian confession, then, leads to the same psychological liberation as do the best psychoanalytical techniques. As I write these lines, I am going over in my mind an interview I had today with a Sister of Charity

51

whom I shall call Florence. She had been sent to me by her superior.

Without any preamble she admitted that her difficulty was that she did not know how to begin to tell me about the problems on her mind. So we began with some small-talk about her work. She is scrupulous, shy, gloomy, full of worries, especially about her work, at which she is too slow. Her state of mind is a further worry to her, bebause she feels she is being a bad witness to Christ by being so lacking in joy. Then she has doubts about her vocation—doubts which take away the last positive prop on which she might lean. This vicious circle of thought has made her ill. Her superiors have already transferred her once to other work, but without securing improvement.

I say hardly anything. Her story goes, bit by bit, right back to the sources of her vocation, then to her childhood memories, to the premature death of her mother, and the moral barries which separated her from her father. Then, all at once, she goes to a deeper level still. While I pray in silence, she tells of terrible emotional shocks suffered in childhood, which have weighed on her mind all her life. I cannot of course recount them here, but what I want to point out is that they are the sort of repressed memories which psychoanalytical technique sometimes helps to bring out into the daylight, but never as quickly as this.

When I thanked Florence for the trust she had shown in me by being so frank, she replied simply that what had made it possible was that she had come with me into the presence of God.

I then suggested to her that she should pray, to bring all these things from her past and lay them at the foot of the Cross. But she did not dare to pray aloud—and this too was a great obstacle to her in her service for Christ. After some minutes of silence, however, she found the courage to make this second decisive step. When she left my consulting room she was radiant, and had no further doubts about her vocation.

Early one Sunday morning my wife asked me to take the dog out. I did so, but I was protesting inwardly. My protest was the assertion of my right to sleep on a Sunday morning! There was also self-pity at having to get up. I went back to bed with these negative thoughts turning over in my mind. The result: I found it impossible to go back to sleep. And the fact that I could not get back to sleep again encouraged my negative thoughts and complaints. All at once I realized that what was stopping me sleeping was not my morning walk, but the complaining thoughts about it that I had allowed to develop in my mind. I saw that I should have got back to sleep long before if my inward complaints had not kept sleep at bay, that I was the victim of my own attitude, and not of circumstances. I went to sleep again at once.

What antagonizes a person is not the truth, but the tone of scorn, pity, criticism, or reproof which so often colors the statement of the truth by those around him. It is that which sets up in him the fear of being cured. A patient once said to me in a letter: "I have to tell you that I am afraid of feeling myself becoming normal. I feel that everyone is going to be taking advantage of me, treating me unkindly. . . . I am defending myself in advance."

To break all these vicious circles, to smash through the chains of cause and effect, what is needed is a confidence strong enough to transcend them, which springs from an experience of God's grace. In the presence of God, in an atmosphere of trust and sincere fellowship, two persons can all at once break free from all the bonds that have been determining their attitude to each other, and have the courage both to see clearly into their own souls and to allow themselves to be seen as clearly.

The Field of Consciousness and Realism

The theory of the contraction of the field of consciousness, which we owe to Pierre Janet, and which has been developed by the psychoanalytical school, provides the best explanation of neurosis. These psychologists have shown that when a deep-seated tendency opposed to the moral ideal of the subject makes its presence felt within him, or shows itself through actions of which his conscience disapproves, the memory of these guilty feelings or acts is driven out of the field of consciousness. Later these repressed tendencies and memories reappear, disguised in the form of mental pictures, dreams, bungled actions, or else as neurotic symptoms, paralyses, functional disorders, obsessions, and so on.

This doctrine can be seen to be in full accord with Christian teaching on the human personality. The only difference is that Christianity calls these "deep-seated tendencies opposed to the moral ideal of the subject" simply sin. The Bible shows that man naturally tends to shut his eyes to his faults and to his sufferings. He tends to eliminate from the field of his consciousness any thoughts, memories, events, or temptations connect-

54

ed ·with sin. Christ, quoting the words of the prophet Isaiah, speaks of the eyes which do not see, the ears which do not hear, and the hearts which do not understand (Mark 8:17-18). The contraction of the field of consciousness could hardly be more clearly described.

The better a man succeeds in becoming honest with himself, the more clearly he will see his field of consciousness will expand. When a man meditates in the presence of God, he learns once more how to look his faults in the face. There takes place within him an expansion of the field of consciousness comparable to that obtained by Janet using hypnosis, and by Freud using the analysis of dreams and bungled actions. In Christian soul-healing I always feel that I am accompanying my patient on a tour of his mind. He ventures into it as into a darkened room: At first nothing is visible, and then gradually one begins to make out shapeless masses—particular problems, one presumes. Slowly these masses loom up out of the darkness, take on more definite outlines, begin to show more and more detail, until, by the light of Jesus Christ, the mind is known.

Science studies man from without. Meditation reveals him from within. We see then how often the conscious and the unconscious counterbalance each other; a conscious virtue hides an unconscious failing. We find that the true motives of our behavior are less flattering than we think, and we see that we are the brothers of all sinners and of all the sick. We discover that in ourselves there are repressed ideas, pretenses, deceit, and fears just like those of our patients, and we can help them then to free themselves from them. I strike my dog bebause he has been disobedient. But when I consider this during my meditation, I realize that in reality I was annoyed with my wife because of a remark she had made to me, and which at the time I pretended to accept, when in fact I had not accepted it. As soon as I make this discovery and write it down in my notebook, or tell my wife about it and ask her to forgive me, I perceive that I already knew of it, but did not dare to admit it clearly to myself. Meditation was needed before I could become aware of what I already knew.

Those who find meditation hardest to practice are the intellectuals. They are assailed by doubts, and wonder if their thoughts are coming from God; whereas a manual laborer, for example, will set down right away on his paper everything that comes into his mind. Then he sees that it is so true, so concrete, and so forthright that he cannot doubt that it comes from God.

Similarly, in meditation, among the thousands of possible associations of ideas, God guides our minds toward certain associations which our complexes (that is to say, our sin) would have prevented us making in any other circumstances. There is therefore no contradiction between psychological determinism and guidance by God of the mind in meditation.

Meditation is thought guided by God. Nothing is better for the mind than a few days spent in solitude and devoted entirely to meditation and to the pooling of thoughts discovered in this way. My wife and I have done this several times. It is the best kind of holiday, the most luminous days it is possible to live through. It is also the profoundest way for a married couple to get to know each other.

True love often makes us see in those we love failings we never noticed when we did not care about them. And so we must go back to what Jesus said. He does not deny that there is a speck in our brother's eye, nor that it may be a charitable act to try and get it out for him. He simply tells us to consider first the log in our own eye; that it to say, to direct the searchlight of our field of consciousness upon ourselves. The more clearly we learn to see our own faults, the freer shall we be from the spirit of criticism.

Thus through the repentance and forgiveness to which it leads, Christian soul-healing provides the answer to all the disorders of the field of consciousness: contraction, expansion in respect of other people, expansion in respect of oneself, and displacement.

But it brings furthermore a quite different kind of succor to the troubled mind, a succor whose effect is synthesis. I have mentioned the danger of overdoing self-analysis. The safeguard against this danger is the Christian vocation of which I shall be speaking in the next chapter. "Overcome evil with good," writes St. Paul (Rom. 12:21), and in doing so he invites those who are getting lost in the labyrinth of self-analysis to turn their eyes away toward the positive call of the gospel of Jesus Christ.

"Forgetting what lies behind, and straining forward to what lies ahead, I press on toward the goal," writes St. Paul again (Phil. 3:13-14). Conscious of God's forgiveness, the mind, without going analytically into all the remote factors in its difficulties, can resolve them all by making the leap of faith. It abandons the fruitless search into the past, and the empty analysis of the present, and can turn its thoughts toward action.

In the practice of spiritual meditation one becomes able to see clearly into one's own mind, but one also learns to see more clearly what it is that God is expecting one to do. A young man once told me of a conversation he had had the day before with a friend. As he was speaking to him about looking for God's will in meditation, his friend interrupted him with these words: "What you call God, I call my conscience."

"Our conscience tells us what we must not do," the young man replied, "but God tells us what we must do."

God has a plan for each one of us. He has prepared us for it by means of the particular gifts and temperament he has given to each of us. To discern this plan through seeking day by day to know his will is to find the purpose of our lives. Having an aim in life is a fundamental condition of physical, moral, and spiritual health.

The world desperately needs people who have a firm conviction of their vocation. When one asks people about what it was that determined their choice of career, one is surprised to find that very many have no clear idea. Others admit to having acted on lesser motives—the hope of earning a living more easily, obedience to a family prejudice, a more or less naive admiration for an elder brother or sister. The man who receives his vocation from God brings a quite different conviction to it. God's purpose for society is realized by men who take up in it the positions that God has prepared for them, and for which he has fitted them through the talents with which he has endowed them. They are possibly more modest places than could have been secured for them by the intervention of their influential uncles. But the people will be happier and more useful in them.

A conviction of vocation—any vocation—is a real motive force in a person's life, ensuring full physical development, psychic equilibrium, and more useful in them.

A man who has decided to submit his life to God's authority does not look to him for guidance only when he has some great decision to make, such as the choice of a career or a wife. Day by day he finds in meditation fresh inspiration for his daily work, his personal behavior, and his attitude toward those about him. I have given a number of examples of this in the course of this book. My experience is that when God's guidance is sought in this way, those conditions of life which are most favorable to health are gradually established. We still make frequent mistakes over what God is expecting of us; we often take our own inclinations for a divine call; we still frequently disobey. And yet if we remain loyal we become more and more able to see our own errors, and more faithful in correcting them.

A diet governed by God, and not by gluttony or fashion; sleep, rest, and holidays dictated by God, and not by laziness or selfishness; a career, work, and physical recreation guided by God, and not by ambition or fear; a sex life, marriage, and family life directed by God, and not by the desire for personal gratification or by jealousy; personal discipline in the use of our time, in imagination and thoughts, imposed by God and not by caprice or the need to escape—these are the fundamental conditions of health both physical and psychical.

The Bible is mainly the story of men who believed in the will of God, who sought to know and to follow it even in the smallest details of their personal life. It shows us men who knew how to listen to God's voice and obey him, who sought to know what God wanted them to say, where he wanted them to go, and what he wanted them to do. All the books of the Prophets, and that of the Acts of the Apostles, are but pictures of men's lives guided by God. The Gospels recount the completely guided life of Jesus Christ. They show him meditating and fasting in the desert, fighting against the temptations of the Devil, and seeking God's inspiration for his ministry. They show him going away by himself in the early morning to meet God face to face and receive his orders for the day's work. They show him constantly escaping from the flattery of men and their worldly requests, to continue on his way from place to place, in accordance with God's plan. They show him, on the eve of the Passion, withdrawing with his disciples, at Caesarea Philippi, and hearing God's call to go up to Jerusalem to suffer and to die there, and telling his disciples of his decision. They show him in the Garden of Gethsemane, still seeking to follow God's will rather than his own.

And throughout the church's history, all the saints who have exerted a profound influence on humanity have been men and women who, breaking away from the conventions of society, and even from the customs of church people, have obeyed God's commands—commands which their contemporaries often failed to understand.

There are countless doctors who look upon their vocation as a social priesthood, and who, in remote valleys or in the slums of our great cities, give themselves unstintingly in the fight against the sufferings of mankind. I am very far from disregarding all their noble zeal and all their disinterested charity. It is to them that I speak. Believers or not, they live in the shadow of Christ. But they occupy an observation post that is particularly well placed for seeing the sufferings that are heaped upon humanity by sin. And, like me, they know that sin creeps craftily into the most dedicated of lives, and the struggle is a hard one. Like me, they know that the materialism which has dominated medicine for a century has not helped us in this struggle against ourselves. Like me, they know that on their personal victory depend the moral victories of their patients, that on the quality of their personal lives depends the beneficent effect they will have on the lives of many a family. And they often feel lonely, discouraged, and overwhelmed.

They are saddened by some of the trends observable in the way our profession is developing, its moral decline, the ravages wrought by the lust for monetary gain which has been denounced in several excellent books. They are well aware that there will be no real amendment of this situation apart from a spiritual renewal in the soul of the doctor. The artisans of this amendment will be doctors who accept the sovereignty of Jesus Christ.

The Christian life does not consist in being perfect, much less in claiming to be so. On the contrary, it consists in being honest about one's shortcomings so as to be able to turn to Jesus Christ for forgiveness and liberation.

I cannot conclude a book in which I have shown the favorable consequences to health of a specifically Christian experience without touching upon a question which more than one reader, no doubt, would like to put to me: "May there not be unfavorable consequences? Are there not some mental disorders which are actually brought about by a religious experience? Are not some patients who believe they have had a spiritual experience of this kind simply the victims of mental disorders?" Yes, of course; that is incontestable. I side unequivocally with the Rev. Fr. De Sinéty, who maintains that no greater disservice can be done to the cause of Christianity than to deny that pathological disorders can simulate genuine religious experience. But he points out that the fact that there are pseudo-mystics does not give us the right to deny that there are real ones.

The same is true of miraculous cures, which I have intentionally bypassed, because they are rather a special case among the subjects that have a bearing on the relationship between medicine and religion. We have no right to deny that miraculous cures do sometimes take place, simply because a large number that are claimed as miraculous can be shown to be merely the result of psychological suggestion.

Finally, it is only right for me to say that I could report several cases where I have been called upon to deal with serious mental disorders that have made their appearance following religious experiences, particularly meetings for witness. I have several times had to have such people sent to mental institutions.

Spiritual power is the greatest power in the world. Although, in order to shake a person out of his state of self-satisfaction, make him look at himself properly, and draw him out of the fortress of compromise in which he has taken refuge from an unquiet conscience, it is often necessary to subject him to the intense emotion of long spiritual retreats, this same power can in others spark serious mental accidents. Such accidents are in fact a proof of the power of the spiritual, just as medicinal intoxication is a proof of the pharmaco-dynamics of medicines. All around us there are people whose psychological equilibrium is so unstable that they are ready to burst out at any moment. Any emotional shock can spark off the conflagration: bereavement, being thwarted, even a physical disease. It is not surprising therefore that experiences touching on a subject as emotionally charged as religion should also be capable of provoking it.

Does this mean that neurotics ought to be kept away from the message of Christianity? What I said just now about the pharmaco-dynamics of medicines seems to me to provide the answer to this question. The same message which when delivered too abruptly and wholesale may provoke mental disorders, may also, when given in proper doses, be a healing agent. The unstable equilibrium of a person with neurotic tendencies is made up of countless compromises; nevertheless it is an equilibrium. A total decision for Christ is capable of producing a better equilibrium. But such a decision first reopens so many unresolved problems that there is a critical zone to cross.

To be religious one does not have to be simple-minded. It does not help neurotics if we are taken in by their facile spiritual enthusiasms. Charity demands that we be severe and realistic with neurotics, that we should always be bringing them back to the concrete problems of their lives, that we should not be content with anything but a patient effort to solve these problems, denouncing every unconcious attempt to escape in the direction of some easy mystical mirage, and helping them to put into practice, little by little, each new glimpse of God's will for them. There are many people—both among believers and among those who use this as an argument against the Christian faith—who make the mistake of thinking that the Christian must necessarily be naïve. Jesus showed himself a true realist when he said that his disciples would be recognizable not by what they said but by the quality of their lives, like a tree by its fruit. We betray the spiritual cause if we allow ourselves to be deceived by people who think their lives have changed because their state of mind has changed, without any real fruit being borne in their daily lives. I could record here many sad cases of neuropaths, especially those of cycloid personality type, who, following upon a theological discussion with a believer—very frequently belonging to one of the Protestant sects—have thought they "understood everything," and have made much of a "conversion" which actually has been purely intellectual. What in fact has happened is that their humor has oscillated from pessimism to optimism, but it is as unreal as it was before. I do not question their sincerity, nor that of those who have communicated to them their theological thoughts. But with those who suffer from nervous disorders one cannot be too realistic, nor too severe in demanding that every new discovery in the realm of the spirit be accompanied by concrete acts of obedience. When one has oneself experienced conversion, one knows what inner battles are involved. One no longer underestimates sin's powers of resistance, and one stresses that the Christian answer is the most costly of all.

I am reminded of one of my patients whose life was a skein of problems of all kinds. In our very first interview she told me that she wanted to follow the way of the Christian life. I told her at once that such a decision was valueless and would only lead to disappointments unless she undertook at once courageously to measure the full consequences of it. And I sent her, that same day, to see a young woman who had the patience to devote her whole time to her for four days running, until my patient had written the letters of apology and put into effect the practical decisions necessary to create a new climate in her life.

Faith is not a matter of feeling. For fear of seeming neurotic, many people refrain all their lives from making any affirmation of their faith. They are afraid of religious psychosis. They are afraid of becoming enthusiastic only to be disillusioned later on.

They have not yet realized that true Christianity does not in fact consist of unreal flights of fancy, but of quite concrete experiences.

There are three roads in front of every man: reality without God, which is the dissociation of the materialists; God without reality, which is the dissociation of the pseudo-mystics; and, lastly, God with reality, which is the Christian faith.

This last is the hardest of the three. For it is far easier to live life as we find it, remaining deaf to God's call; or else to answer his call sentimentally, while closing one's eyes to reality. It is easier to be either a materialist or an idealist. What is difficult is to be a Christian.

I come back here to the point from which I started this book, that men's lives are full of concrete problems, material as well as psychological. A religious conversion which avoids these problems, leaving them unresolved, is what too often brings Christianity into disrepute. But a conversion which brings the solution of the problems in a person's life is a living proof of the power of Christ.